RATING
☆☆☆☆☆

PREP TIME

COOKING TIME

DIFFICULTY
○○○○○

SOURCE

NUMBER OF SERVINGS

1 2 3 4 5 ....

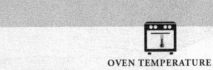

OVEN TEMPERATURE

°C

INGREDIENTS

METHOD

NOTES

RECIPE ORIGIN

RATING

PREP TIME

COOKING TIME

DIFFICULTY

SOURCE

OVEN TEMPERATURE

NUMBER OF SERVINGS

1 2 3 4 5 ....

°C

INGREDIENTS

METHOD

NOTES

RECIPE ORIGIN

RATING
☆☆☆☆☆

PREP TIME

SOURCE

NUMBER OF SERVINGS

1 2 3 4 5 ....

INGREDIENTS

RECIPE ORIGIN

COOKING TIME

DIFFICULTY
○○○○○

OVEN TEMPERATURE

°C

NOTES

METHOD

RATING
☆☆☆☆☆

PREP TIME

COOKING TIME

DIFFICULTY

SOURCE

OVEN TEMPERATURE

NUMBER OF SERVINGS

1 2 3 4 5 ....

INGREDIENTS

METHOD

NOTES

RECIPE ORIGIN

RATING
☆☆☆☆☆

PREP TIME

COOKING TIME

DIFFICULTY

OVEN TEMPERATURE

SOURCE

NUMBER OF SERVINGS

1 2 3 4 5 ....

INGREDIENTS

METHOD

NOTES

RECIPE ORIGIN

RATING
☆☆☆☆☆

PREP TIME

COOKING TIME

DIFFICULTY

SOURCE

OVEN TEMPERATURE
°C

NUMBER OF SERVINGS

1 2 3 4 5 ....

INGREDIENTS

_____
_____
_____
_____
_____
_____
_____

NOTES

_____
_____
_____
_____

RECIPE ORIGIN

METHOD

_____
_____
_____
_____
_____
_____
_____
_____
_____
_____
_____
_____
_____
_____

RATING

☆☆☆☆☆

PREP TIME

COOKING TIME

DIFFICULTY

SOURCE

OVEN TEMPERATURE

NUMBER OF SERVINGS

1 2 3 4 5 ....

INGREDIENTS

METHOD

NOTES

RECIPE ORIGIN

RATING
☆☆☆☆☆

PREP TIME

COOKING TIME

DIFFICULTY

SOURCE

OVEN TEMPERATURE
°C

NUMBER OF SERVINGS
1 2 3 4 5 ....

INGREDIENTS

NOTES

METHOD

RECIPE ORIGIN

RATING
☆☆☆☆☆

PREP TIME

COOKING TIME

DIFFICULTY

OVEN TEMPERATURE

SOURCE

NUMBER OF SERVINGS

1 2 3 4 5 ....

INGREDIENTS

METHOD

NOTES

RECIPE ORIGIN

RATING
☆☆☆☆☆

PREP TIME

SOURCE

NUMBER OF SERVINGS

1 2 3 4 5 ....

INGREDIENTS

_____
_____
_____
_____
_____
_____
_____

RECIPE ORIGIN

COOKING TIME

DIFFICULTY
○○○○○

OVEN TEMPERATURE
_____ °C

NOTES
_____
_____
_____
_____
_____
_____
_____

METHOD

_____
_____
_____
_____
_____
_____
_____
_____
_____
_____
_____
_____
_____
_____

RATING
☆☆☆☆☆

PREP TIME

SOURCE

NUMBER OF SERVINGS

1 2 3 4 5 ....

INGREDIENTS

RECIPE ORIGIN

COOKING TIME

DIFFICULTY
○○○○○

OVEN TEMPERATURE

°C

NOTES

METHOD

RATING
☆☆☆☆☆

PREP TIME

COOKING TIME

DIFFICULTY

OVEN TEMPERATURE

SOURCE

NUMBER OF SERVINGS

1 2 3 4 5 ....

INGREDIENTS

METHOD

NOTES

RECIPE ORIGIN

RATING
☆☆☆☆☆

PREP TIME
:

COOKING TIME

DIFFICULTY
○○○○

SOURCE

OVEN TEMPERATURE
°C

NUMBER OF SERVINGS

1 2 3 4 5 ....

INGREDIENTS

METHOD

NOTES

RECIPE ORIGIN

RATING
☆☆☆☆☆

PREP TIME

COOKING TIME

DIFFICULTY

SOURCE

OVEN TEMPERATURE

NUMBER OF SERVINGS

1 2 3 4 5 ....

°C

INGREDIENTS

METHOD

NOTES

RECIPE ORIGIN

RATING
☆☆☆☆☆

PREP TIME
:

COOKING TIME

DIFFICULTY

SOURCE

OVEN TEMPERATURE

NUMBER OF SERVINGS
1 2 3 4 5 ....

INGREDIENTS

METHOD

NOTES

RECIPE ORIGIN

RATING
☆☆☆☆☆

PREP TIME

SOURCE

NUMBER OF SERVINGS

1 2 3 4 5 ....

INGREDIENTS

RECIPE ORIGIN

COOKING TIME

DIFFICULTY

OVEN TEMPERATURE

°C

METHOD

NOTES

RATING
☆☆☆☆☆

PREP TIME

SOURCE

NUMBER OF SERVINGS

1 2 3 4 5 ....

INGREDIENTS

COOKING TIME

DIFFICULTY
○○○○○

OVEN TEMPERATURE

°C

METHOD

NOTES

RECIPE ORIGIN

RATING
☆☆☆☆☆

PREP TIME

COOKING TIME

DIFFICULTY

SOURCE

OVEN TEMPERATURE

NUMBER OF SERVINGS

1 2 3 4 5 ....

INGREDIENTS

METHOD

NOTES

RECIPE ORIGIN

RATING
☆☆☆☆☆

PREP TIME

COOKING TIME

DIFFICULTY
○○○○○

SOURCE

OVEN TEMPERATURE

NUMBER OF SERVINGS

1 2 3 4 5 ....

°C

INGREDIENTS

METHOD

NOTES

RECIPE ORIGIN

RATING
☆☆☆☆☆

PREP TIME

SOURCE

NUMBER OF SERVINGS

1 2 3 4 5 ....

INGREDIENTS

RECIPE ORIGIN

COOKING TIME

DIFFICULTY

OVEN TEMPERATURE

°C

METHOD

NOTES

RATING
☆☆☆☆☆

PREP TIME

COOKING TIME

DIFFICULTY

SOURCE

OVEN TEMPERATURE

NUMBER OF SERVINGS

1 2 3 4 5 ....

°C

INGREDIENTS

METHOD

NOTES

RECIPE ORIGIN

RATING
☆☆☆☆☆

PREP TIME

COOKING TIME

DIFFICULTY

OVEN TEMPERATURE
°C

SOURCE

NUMBER OF SERVINGS
1 2 3 4 5 ....

INGREDIENTS

METHOD

NOTES

RECIPE ORIGIN

RATING
☆☆☆☆☆

PREP TIME

SOURCE

NUMBER OF SERVINGS

1 2 3 4 5 ....

COOKING TIME

DIFFICULTY

OVEN TEMPERATURE

°C

INGREDIENTS

_____
_____
_____
_____
_____
_____
_____

RECIPE ORIGIN

NOTES

METHOD

_____
_____
_____
_____
_____
_____
_____
_____
_____
_____
_____
_____
_____

RATING
☆☆☆☆☆

PREP TIME

COOKING TIME

DIFFICULTY

SOURCE

OVEN TEMPERATURE

NUMBER OF SERVINGS
1 2 3 4 5 ....

°C

INGREDIENTS

METHOD

NOTES

RECIPE ORIGIN

RATING
☆☆☆☆☆

PREP TIME

COOKING TIME

DIFFICULTY

OVEN TEMPERATURE

SOURCE

NUMBER OF SERVINGS

1 2 3 4 5 ....

INGREDIENTS

METHOD

NOTES

RECIPE ORIGIN

RATING
☆☆☆☆☆

PREP TIME

COOKING TIME

DIFFICULTY

SOURCE

OVEN TEMPERATURE

NUMBER OF SERVINGS

1 2 3 4 5 ....

INGREDIENTS

METHOD

NOTES

RECIPE ORIGIN

RATING
☆☆☆☆☆

PREP TIME

COOKING TIME

DIFFICULTY

SOURCE

OVEN TEMPERATURE

NUMBER OF SERVINGS

1 2 3 4 5 ....

°C

INGREDIENTS

METHOD

NOTES

RECIPE ORIGIN

RATING
☆☆☆☆☆

PREP TIME

COOKING TIME

DIFFICULTY

SOURCE

OVEN TEMPERATURE

NUMBER OF SERVINGS

1 2 3 4 5 ....

INGREDIENTS

METHOD

NOTES

RECIPE ORIGIN

RATING

☆☆☆☆☆

....

PREP TIME

COOKING TIME

DIFFICULTY
○○○○

SOURCE

OVEN TEMPERATURE

NUMBER OF SERVINGS

1 2 3 4 5 ....

°C

INGREDIENTS

_____
_____
_____
_____
_____
_____
_____

METHOD

_____
_____
_____
_____
_____
_____
_____
_____
_____
_____
_____
_____
_____

NOTES

_____
_____
_____
_____
_____
_____

RECIPE ORIGIN

RATING
☆☆☆☆☆

PREP TIME

COOKING TIME

DIFFICULTY
○○○○○

SOURCE

OVEN TEMPERATURE

NUMBER OF SERVINGS

1 2 3 4 5 ....

°C

INGREDIENTS

METHOD

NOTES

RECIPE ORIGIN

RATING
☆☆☆☆☆

PREP TIME

COOKING TIME

DIFFICULTY

SOURCE

OVEN TEMPERATURE

NUMBER OF SERVINGS

1 2 3 4 5 ....

°C

INGREDIENTS

METHOD

NOTES

RECIPE ORIGIN

RATING
☆☆☆☆☆

PREP TIME

COOKING TIME

DIFFICULTY

SOURCE

OVEN TEMPERATURE

NUMBER OF SERVINGS

1 2 3 4 5 ....

INGREDIENTS

METHOD

NOTES

RECIPE ORIGIN

°C

RATING
☆☆☆☆☆

PREP TIME

COOKING TIME

DIFFICULTY

SOURCE

OVEN TEMPERATURE

NUMBER OF SERVINGS

1 2 3 4 5 ....

°C

INGREDIENTS

METHOD

NOTES

RECIPE ORIGIN

RATING
☆☆☆☆☆

PREP TIME

COOKING TIME

DIFFICULTY

SOURCE

OVEN TEMPERATURE

NUMBER OF SERVINGS

1 2 3 4 5 ....

INGREDIENTS

METHOD

NOTES

RECIPE ORIGIN

RATING
☆☆☆☆☆

PREP TIME

COOKING TIME

DIFFICULTY

OVEN TEMPERATURE

SOURCE

NUMBER OF SERVINGS

1 2 3 4 5 ....

INGREDIENTS

METHOD

NOTES

RECIPE ORIGIN

RATING
☆☆☆☆☆

PREP TIME
:

COOKING TIME

DIFFICULTY
○○○○○

SOURCE

OVEN TEMPERATURE
°C

NUMBER OF SERVINGS
1 2 3 4 5 ....

INGREDIENTS

METHOD

NOTES

RECIPE ORIGIN

RATING
☆☆☆☆☆

PREP TIME

COOKING TIME

DIFFICULTY

OVEN TEMPERATURE

SOURCE

NUMBER OF SERVINGS

1 2 3 4 5 ....

INGREDIENTS

METHOD

NOTES

RECIPE ORIGIN

RATING
☆☆☆☆☆

PREP TIME

COOKING TIME

DIFFICULTY

SOURCE

OVEN TEMPERATURE

NUMBER OF SERVINGS

1 2 3 4 5 ....

INGREDIENTS

METHOD

NOTES

RECIPE ORIGIN

RATING
☆☆☆☆☆

PREP TIME

COOKING TIME

DIFFICULTY

OVEN TEMPERATURE

SOURCE

NUMBER OF SERVINGS

1 2 3 4 5 ....

INGREDIENTS

METHOD

NOTES

RECIPE ORIGIN

RATING
☆☆☆☆☆

PREP TIME

COOKING TIME

DIFFICULTY

SOURCE

OVEN TEMPERATURE

NUMBER OF SERVINGS

1 2 3 4 5 ....

°C

INGREDIENTS

METHOD

NOTES

RECIPE ORIGIN

RATING
☆☆☆☆☆

PREP TIME

COOKING TIME

DIFFICULTY

SOURCE

OVEN TEMPERATURE

NUMBER OF SERVINGS

1 2 3 4 5 ....

INGREDIENTS

METHOD

NOTES

RECIPE ORIGIN

RATING
☆☆☆☆☆

PREP TIME

COOKING TIME

DIFFICULTY

SOURCE

OVEN TEMPERATURE

NUMBER OF SERVINGS

1 2 3 4 5 ....

INGREDIENTS

METHOD

NOTES

RECIPE ORIGIN

RATING
☆☆☆☆☆

PREP TIME

SOURCE

NUMBER OF SERVINGS

1 2 3 4 5 ....

INGREDIENTS

RECIPE ORIGIN

COOKING TIME

DIFFICULTY

OVEN TEMPERATURE
°C

METHOD

NOTES

RATING
☆☆☆☆☆

PREP TIME

COOKING TIME

DIFFICULTY

OVEN TEMPERATURE

SOURCE

NUMBER OF SERVINGS

1 2 3 4 5 ....

INGREDIENTS

METHOD

NOTES

RECIPE ORIGIN

RATING
☆☆☆☆☆

PREP TIME

COOKING TIME

DIFFICULTY

SOURCE

OVEN TEMPERATURE

NUMBER OF SERVINGS

1 2 3 4 5 ....

°C

INGREDIENTS

METHOD

NOTES

RECIPE ORIGIN

RATING
☆☆☆☆☆

PREP TIME

COOKING TIME

DIFFICULTY

SOURCE

OVEN TEMPERATURE

NUMBER OF SERVINGS

1 2 3 4 5 ....

INGREDIENTS

METHOD

NOTES

RECIPE ORIGIN

RATING
☆☆☆☆☆

....

PREP TIME

COOKING TIME

DIFFICULTY

SOURCE

OVEN TEMPERATURE

NUMBER OF SERVINGS

1 2 3 4 5 ....

°C

INGREDIENTS

METHOD

NOTES

RECIPE ORIGIN

RATING
☆☆☆☆☆

PREP TIME

COOKING TIME

DIFFICULTY

SOURCE

OVEN TEMPERATURE

NUMBER OF SERVINGS

1 2 3 4 5 ....

INGREDIENTS

NOTES

METHOD

RECIPE ORIGIN

RATING
☆☆☆☆☆

PREP TIME

COOKING TIME

DIFFICULTY

OVEN TEMPERATURE

SOURCE

NUMBER OF SERVINGS

1 2 3 4 5 ....

INGREDIENTS

METHOD

NOTES

RECIPE ORIGIN

RATING
☆☆☆☆☆

PREP TIME

COOKING TIME

DIFFICULTY

SOURCE

OVEN TEMPERATURE

NUMBER OF SERVINGS

1 2 3 4 5 ....

INGREDIENTS

METHOD

NOTES

RECIPE ORIGIN

RATING
☆☆☆☆☆

PREP TIME

COOKING TIME

DIFFICULTY

SOURCE

OVEN TEMPERATURE

NUMBER OF SERVINGS

1 2 3 4 5 ....

INGREDIENTS

METHOD

NOTES

RECIPE ORIGIN

RATING

☆☆☆☆☆

PREP TIME

COOKING TIME

DIFFICULTY

OVEN TEMPERATURE

°C

SOURCE

NUMBER OF SERVINGS

1 2 3 4 5 ....

INGREDIENTS

METHOD

NOTES

RECIPE ORIGIN

RATING
☆☆☆☆☆

PREP TIME

COOKING TIME

DIFFICULTY
○○○○○

SOURCE

OVEN TEMPERATURE

NUMBER OF SERVINGS

1 2 3 4 5 ....

INGREDIENTS

METHOD

NOTES

RECIPE ORIGIN

RATING
☆☆☆☆☆

PREP TIME

COOKING TIME

DIFFICULTY

SOURCE

OVEN TEMPERATURE

NUMBER OF SERVINGS

1 2 3 4 5 ....

INGREDIENTS

METHOD

NOTES

RECIPE ORIGIN

RATING
☆☆☆☆☆

PREP TIME

SOURCE

NUMBER OF SERVINGS
1 2 3 4 5 ....

COOKING TIME

DIFFICULTY
○○○○○

OVEN TEMPERATURE
°C

INGREDIENTS

METHOD

NOTES

RECIPE ORIGIN

RATING
☆☆☆☆☆

PREP TIME

COOKING TIME

DIFFICULTY

SOURCE

OVEN TEMPERATURE
°C

NUMBER OF SERVINGS
1 2 3 4 5 ....

INGREDIENTS

METHOD

NOTES

RECIPE ORIGIN

RATING
☆☆☆☆☆

PREP TIME

COOKING TIME

DIFFICULTY

OVEN TEMPERATURE

SOURCE

NUMBER OF SERVINGS

1 2 3 4 5 ....

°C

INGREDIENTS

METHOD

NOTES

RECIPE ORIGIN

RATING
☆☆☆☆☆

PREP TIME

SOURCE

NUMBER OF SERVINGS

1 2 3 4 5 ....

INGREDIENTS

RECIPE ORIGIN

COOKING TIME

DIFFICULTY

OVEN TEMPERATURE

°C

NOTES

METHOD

RATING
☆☆☆☆☆

....

PREP TIME
:

COOKING TIME

DIFFICULTY

SOURCE

OVEN TEMPERATURE

NUMBER OF SERVINGS

1 2 3 4 5 ....

°C

INGREDIENTS

METHOD

NOTES

RECIPE ORIGIN

RATING
☆☆☆☆☆

PREP TIME

COOKING TIME

DIFFICULTY

SOURCE

OVEN TEMPERATURE

NUMBER OF SERVINGS

1 2 3 4 5 ....

INGREDIENTS

METHOD

NOTES

RECIPE ORIGIN

RATING
☆☆☆☆☆

....

COOKING TIME

DIFFICULTY
○○○○○

PREP TIME

SOURCE

OVEN TEMPERATURE

NUMBER OF SERVINGS

1 2 3 4 5 ....

INGREDIENTS

METHOD

NOTES

RECIPE ORIGIN

RATING
☆☆☆☆☆

PREP TIME

COOKING TIME

DIFFICULTY

SOURCE

OVEN TEMPERATURE

NUMBER OF SERVINGS

1 2 3 4 5 ....

°C

INGREDIENTS

METHOD

NOTES

RECIPE ORIGIN

RATING
☆☆☆☆☆

PREP TIME

COOKING TIME

DIFFICULTY
○○○○○

SOURCE

OVEN TEMPERATURE
°C

NUMBER OF SERVINGS
1 2 3 4 5 ....

INGREDIENTS

_____
_____
_____
_____
_____
_____
_____
_____

METHOD

_____
_____
_____
_____
_____
_____
_____
_____
_____
_____
_____
_____

NOTES

_____
_____
_____
_____
_____

RECIPE ORIGIN

RATING
☆☆☆☆☆

PREP TIME

COOKING TIME

DIFFICULTY

OVEN TEMPERATURE

SOURCE

NUMBER OF SERVINGS

1 2 3 4 5 ....

INGREDIENTS

METHOD

NOTES

RECIPE ORIGIN

RATING
☆☆☆☆☆

....

PREP TIME
:

COOKING TIME

DIFFICULTY
○○○○○

SOURCE

OVEN TEMPERATURE

°C

NUMBER OF SERVINGS

1 2 3 4 5 ....

INGREDIENTS

METHOD

NOTES

RECIPE ORIGIN

RATING
☆☆☆☆☆

PREP TIME

COOKING TIME

DIFFICULTY

SOURCE

OVEN TEMPERATURE

NUMBER OF SERVINGS
1 2 3 4 5 ....

INGREDIENTS

METHOD

NOTES

RECIPE ORIGIN

RATING
☆☆☆☆☆

PREP TIME :

COOKING TIME

DIFFICULTY

SOURCE

OVEN TEMPERATURE

NUMBER OF SERVINGS

1 2 3 4 5 ....

°C

INGREDIENTS

METHOD

NOTES

RECIPE ORIGIN

RATING
☆☆☆☆☆

PREP TIME

COOKING TIME

DIFFICULTY

SOURCE

OVEN TEMPERATURE

NUMBER OF SERVINGS

1 2 3 4 5 ....

°C

INGREDIENTS

METHOD

NOTES

RECIPE ORIGIN

RATING
☆☆☆☆☆

PREP TIME

COOKING TIME

DIFFICULTY
○○○○○

SOURCE

OVEN TEMPERATURE

NUMBER OF SERVINGS
1 2 3 4 5 ....

INGREDIENTS

METHOD

NOTES

RECIPE ORIGIN

RATING
☆☆☆☆☆

PREP TIME

COOKING TIME

DIFFICULTY

SOURCE

OVEN TEMPERATURE

NUMBER OF SERVINGS

1 2 3 4 5 ....

°C

INGREDIENTS

METHOD

NOTES

RECIPE ORIGIN

RATING
☆☆☆☆☆

PREP TIME

COOKING TIME

DIFFICULTY

SOURCE

OVEN TEMPERATURE

NUMBER OF SERVINGS

1 2 3 4 5 ....

°C

INGREDIENTS

METHOD

NOTES

RECIPE ORIGIN

RATING
☆☆☆☆☆

PREP TIME

COOKING TIME

DIFFICULTY

SOURCE

OVEN TEMPERATURE

NUMBER OF SERVINGS

1 2 3 4 5 ....

INGREDIENTS

METHOD

NOTES

RECIPE ORIGIN

RATING
☆☆☆☆☆

PREP TIME
:

COOKING TIME

DIFFICULTY
○○○○○

OVEN TEMPERATURE

SOURCE

NUMBER OF SERVINGS
1 2 3 4 5 ....

INGREDIENTS

METHOD

NOTES

RECIPE ORIGIN

RATING
☆☆☆☆☆

PREP TIME

COOKING TIME

DIFFICULTY

SOURCE

OVEN TEMPERATURE

NUMBER OF SERVINGS
1 2 3 4 5 ....

INGREDIENTS

METHOD

NOTES

RECIPE ORIGIN

RATING
☆☆☆☆☆

....

PREP TIME

COOKING TIME

DIFFICULTY

SOURCE

OVEN TEMPERATURE

NUMBER OF SERVINGS

1 2 3 4 5 ....

INGREDIENTS

_____
_____
_____
_____
_____
_____
_____

METHOD

_____
_____
_____
_____
_____
_____
_____
_____
_____
_____
_____

NOTES

_____
_____
_____
_____

RECIPE ORIGIN

RATING
☆☆☆☆☆

PREP TIME

COOKING TIME

DIFFICULTY

SOURCE

OVEN TEMPERATURE

NUMBER OF SERVINGS

1 2 3 4 5 ....

°C

INGREDIENTS

METHOD

NOTES

RECIPE ORIGIN

RATING
☆☆☆☆☆

PREP TIME
:

COOKING TIME

DIFFICULTY
○○○○○

SOURCE

OVEN TEMPERATURE

NUMBER OF SERVINGS

1 2 3 4 5 ....

INGREDIENTS

METHOD

NOTES

RECIPE ORIGIN

RATING
☆☆☆☆☆

PREP TIME

SOURCE

NUMBER OF SERVINGS

1 2 3 4 5 ....

INGREDIENTS

RECIPE ORIGIN

COOKING TIME

DIFFICULTY

OVEN TEMPERATURE
°C

NOTES

METHOD

RATING
☆☆☆☆☆

....

PREP TIME

COOKING TIME

DIFFICULTY

SOURCE

OVEN TEMPERATURE

NUMBER OF SERVINGS

1 2 3 4 5 ....

INGREDIENTS

_____
_____
_____
_____
_____
_____
_____
_____

RECIPE ORIGIN

NOTES

_____
_____
_____
_____
_____
_____

METHOD

_____
_____
_____
_____
_____
_____
_____
_____
_____
_____
_____
_____
_____
_____

RATING
☆☆☆☆☆

PREP TIME

COOKING TIME

DIFFICULTY

SOURCE

OVEN TEMPERATURE

NUMBER OF SERVINGS

1 2 3 4 5 ....

INGREDIENTS

METHOD

NOTES

RECIPE ORIGIN

RATING
☆☆☆☆☆

PREP TIME

SOURCE

NUMBER OF SERVINGS

1 2 3 4 5 ....

INGREDIENTS

RECIPE ORIGIN

COOKING TIME

DIFFICULTY

OVEN TEMPERATURE

°C

NOTES

METHOD

RATING
☆☆☆☆☆

PREP TIME

COOKING TIME

DIFFICULTY

OVEN TEMPERATURE

SOURCE

NUMBER OF SERVINGS

1 2 3 4 5 ....

INGREDIENTS

RECIPE ORIGIN

NOTES

METHOD

RATING
☆☆☆☆☆

....

PREP TIME

COOKING TIME

DIFFICULTY

SOURCE

OVEN TEMPERATURE

NUMBER OF SERVINGS

1 2 3 4 5 ....

°C

INGREDIENTS

METHOD

NOTES

RECIPE ORIGIN

RATING
☆☆☆☆☆

:
PREP TIME

COOKING TIME

DIFFICULTY
●●●●●

SOURCE

OVEN TEMPERATURE

NUMBER OF SERVINGS

1 2 3 4 5 ....

°C

INGREDIENTS

METHOD

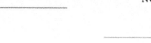
NOTES

RECIPE ORIGIN

RATING
☆☆☆☆☆

....

PREP TIME

COOKING TIME

DIFFICULTY
○○○○

SOURCE

OVEN TEMPERATURE

NUMBER OF SERVINGS

1 2 3 4 5 ....

°C

INGREDIENTS

METHOD

NOTES

RECIPE ORIGIN

RATING
☆☆☆☆☆

PREP TIME

COOKING TIME

DIFFICULTY

SOURCE

OVEN TEMPERATURE

NUMBER OF SERVINGS

1 2 3 4 5 ....

INGREDIENTS

METHOD

NOTES

RECIPE ORIGIN

RATING
☆☆☆☆☆

PREP TIME

COOKING TIME

DIFFICULTY

OVEN TEMPERATURE
°C

SOURCE

NUMBER OF SERVINGS

1 2 3 4 5 ....

INGREDIENTS

METHOD

NOTES

RECIPE ORIGIN

RATING
☆☆☆☆☆

PREP TIME

COOKING TIME

DIFFICULTY

SOURCE

OVEN TEMPERATURE
°C

NUMBER OF SERVINGS

1 2 3 4 5 ....

INGREDIENTS

METHOD

NOTES

RECIPE ORIGIN

RATING
☆☆☆☆☆

PREP TIME

COOKING TIME

DIFFICULTY
○○○○○

SOURCE

OVEN TEMPERATURE

NUMBER OF SERVINGS

1 2 3 4 5 ....

°C

INGREDIENTS

METHOD

NOTES

RECIPE ORIGIN

RATING
☆☆☆☆☆

PREP TIME

COOKING TIME

DIFFICULTY

SOURCE

OVEN TEMPERATURE

NUMBER OF SERVINGS
1 2 3 4 5 ....

°C

INGREDIENTS

METHOD

NOTES

RECIPE ORIGIN

RATING
☆☆☆☆☆

PREP TIME

SOURCE

NUMBER OF SERVINGS

1 2 3 4 5 ....

INGREDIENTS

_____
_____
_____
_____
_____
_____
_____

RECIPE ORIGIN

COOKING TIME

DIFFICULTY

OVEN TEMPERATURE

°C

NOTES

METHOD

RATING
☆☆☆☆☆

PREP TIME

COOKING TIME

DIFFICULTY

SOURCE

OVEN TEMPERATURE

NUMBER OF SERVINGS
1 2 3 4 5 ....

°C

INGREDIENTS

METHOD

NOTES

RECIPE ORIGIN

RATING
☆☆☆☆☆

PREP TIME

COOKING TIME

DIFFICULTY

SOURCE

OVEN TEMPERATURE

NUMBER OF SERVINGS

1 2 3 4 5 ....

°C

INGREDIENTS

METHOD

NOTES

RECIPE ORIGIN

RATING
☆☆☆☆☆

PREP TIME

COOKING TIME

DIFFICULTY

SOURCE

OVEN TEMPERATURE

NUMBER OF SERVINGS

1 2 3 4 5 ....

INGREDIENTS

METHOD

NOTES

RECIPE ORIGIN

RATING
☆☆☆☆☆

PREP TIME

COOKING TIME

DIFFICULTY

SOURCE

OVEN TEMPERATURE

NUMBER OF SERVINGS

1 2 3 4 5 ....

INGREDIENTS

METHOD

NOTES

RECIPE ORIGIN

RATING

PREP TIME

COOKING TIME

DIFFICULTY

SOURCE

OVEN TEMPERATURE

NUMBER OF SERVINGS

1 2 3 4 5 ....

INGREDIENTS

METHOD

NOTES

RECIPE ORIGIN

RATING
☆☆☆☆☆

PREP TIME
:

COOKING TIME

DIFFICULTY
○○○○○

SOURCE

OVEN TEMPERATURE

NUMBER OF SERVINGS

1 2 3 4 5 ....

INGREDIENTS

_____
_____
_____
_____
_____
_____
_____
_____
_____

METHOD

_____
_____
_____
_____
_____
_____
_____
_____
_____
_____
_____
_____
_____

NOTES

_____
_____
_____
_____
_____
_____
_____
_____

RECIPE ORIGIN

RATING
☆☆☆☆☆

PREP TIME

COOKING TIME

DIFFICULTY

OVEN TEMPERATURE

SOURCE

NUMBER OF SERVINGS

1 2 3 4 5 ....

INGREDIENTS

METHOD

NOTES

RECIPE ORIGIN

RATING
☆☆☆☆☆

PREP TIME

SOURCE

NUMBER OF SERVINGS

1 2 3 4 5 ....

INGREDIENTS

_____
_____
_____
_____
_____
_____
_____

RECIPE ORIGIN

COOKING TIME

DIFFICULTY
○○○○○

OVEN TEMPERATURE
°C

METHOD

_____
_____
_____
_____
_____
_____
_____
_____
_____
_____
_____
_____
_____

NOTES

RATING
☆☆☆☆☆

PREP TIME

COOKING TIME

DIFFICULTY

SOURCE

OVEN TEMPERATURE
°C

NUMBER OF SERVINGS
1 2 3 4 5 ....

INGREDIENTS

METHOD

NOTES

RECIPE ORIGIN

CPSIA information can be obtained
at www.ICGtesting.com
Printed in the USA
BVHW012233210720
584272BV00013BA/257